Paramedic Me...
Made Easy

# Paramedic
## Med Math
# Made Easy

Diane Pettway RN, BSN, MS

iUniverse, Inc.
New York   Bloomington

Paramedic Med-Math Made Easy

iUniverse books may be ordered through booksellers or by contacting:

iUniverse
1663 Liberty Drive
Bloomington, IN 47403
www.iuniverse.com
1-800-Authors (1-800-288-4677)

ISBN: 978-0-595-50635-4 (pbk)
ISBN: 978-0-595-61591-9 (ebk)

Printed in the United States of America

*For my family*

*&*

*All the emergency care medical professionals that save lives everyday*

# Contents

# Acknowledgment

I would like to thank my husband, Pat, and my family for making my life and nursing career so meaningful. It has not been easy over the years putting up with the crazy hours and holiday schedules of a nurse. Pat, I also want to thank you for all the endless hours and juggling of schedules so we could raise our beautiful daughter, Amanda, the light of our lives.

# Preface

This book is to assist the out-of-hospital care provider who works in emergency care and has need of good math skills. The material presented will enable the provider to master the skills needed to administer medication using med math formulas. The most commonly used formulas are presented with detailed explanations. Several practice problems have been added at the end of the book. There are also med math practice word problems to prepare you for any exam you may take in med math calculation where no medication labels are in front of you. Answers to the problems and the proper setup of the formulas used to calculate the problems are included.

.

# About the Author

Diane Pettway RN has been a Registered Nurse for more than twenty-six years. She has clinical experience in medical/surgical, critical care, and emergency room nursing as well as experience in nursing management. Diane is currently a full-time assistant professor at a community college, teaching in the paramedic program. She is also an EMT-B and an instructor in ACLS, PALS, ITLS, and BLS.

# Introduction

Welcome to Paramedic Med Math Made Easy. There are many books that cover medication math and all sorts of calculation formulas. This self-help book is a tool that can assist you with studying. You as the student must decide what method works best for you and what will prevent you from making errors in your medication calculations.

Med math does not have to be as hard as you may think. The math presented in this book is commonly used by out-of-hospital care providers.

Paramedic Med Math Made Easy is not a replacement for what you have learned, but it will assist you in using med math to calculate proper dosage of your patients' medications. There are many applications that teach medication calculation; I have not included them all.

The examples in this book are not meant to be used for routine dosing: they are only examples of mathematical calculations with various numbers and doses. The medication labels used in the calculations are only examples and are not meant to be true medication dosing labels.

# Chapter 1
# Equivalents

Before getting into the math calculations, there are some basic math equations that you must know. To start with, let's cover some of the equivalents.

When using math in the medical field, patients are weighed in kilograms (kg). If a patient's weight is in pounds (lbs) you must convert pounds to kilograms. There are 2.2 lbs to every kilogram. Let's see how this works with the following example:

You have a patient who weighs 100 lbs. Take 100 lbs and divide by 2.2 kg. This will give you the correct answer.

$$100 \text{ lbs} \div 2.2 \text{ kgs} = 45.45 \text{ kg}$$

There is another way to figure weight: it is called the 2 a.m. rule. You take the 100 lbs and divide by 2. From that answer (the quotient), subtract 10% of the quotient. The 2 a.m. rule will give you the same answer as the first equation or it will only be off by approximately one pound.

Let's look at the 2 a.m. rule to recalculate the equation:

$$100 lbs \div 2 = 50 \text{ lbs} \quad \text{then} \quad 50 \text{ lbs} \times .10 = 5$$

$$\text{now take} \quad 50 \text{ lbs} - 5 = 45 \text{ kg}$$

When converting weight, you usually round to the nearest whole number. This is how weight will be figured in this book.

The next basic equivalents are for volume:

1 tsp (teaspoon) = 5 ml (milliliters)
1 tbs (tablespoon) = 15 ml
1 oz (ounce) = 30 ml
1 L (liter) = 1000 ml

Now let's look at some basic equivalents for mass:

1 mg (milligram) = 1000 mcg (microgram)
1 gm (gram) = 1000 mg

The equivalent dealing with volume, 1000 ml equals 1 L, is one that is used all the time with intravenous infusions. The other volume equivalents are needed to convert teaspoons, tablespoons, and ounces to milliliters. If a physician orders you to give an oral medication in liquid form to a patient, and the measuring device you have is a syringe marked in milliliters, then you will be able to convert the measurement and give the correct dose. For example, you have an order to give 2 tsp of a liquid medication. Using the syringe you would give 10 ml. If the order was 2 oz, you would give 60 ml. If the order was 2 tbs, you would give 30 ml.

There will be times when you need to change milligrams to micrograms, grams to milligrams, or micrograms to milligrams. This may happen when you have an order for medication to be given in micrograms but you only have a medication vial that measures the drug in milligrams.

*One important action to always remember is never change the physician's order to what you have on hand. Only change what you have on hand to what the physician ordered.*

# Chapter 2
# Formulas

As stated in chapter 1, you only change the drug you have on hand to what the physician ordered. What do I mean by this? The drug you have on hand is the drug available in the medication container that you have in your ambulance and/or in your hand.

Let's look at an example of this:

The physician has ordered you to give a patient 1 gm of a medication intravenously, and the bottle of medication you have is in milligrams. The bottle states that you have 500 mg of drug to every 1 ml. Below is the drug label from the bottle:

```
Drug A

500 mg/ml
```

There are 1000 mg to 1 gm, so 500 mg equals 0.5 gm: this means there are 0.5 gm per 1 ml. You have to convert milligrams to grams. This means you will give 2 ml of this drug to equal the physician's order. When converting milligrams to grams, you just move the decimal point three places to the left. You started with 500, so you will have 0.5 after moving the decimal. Let's look at a formula you can use to get this order correct. The physician's (doctor's) order is to give 1 gm of Drug A, and you have the label on the drug bottle as shown on previous page:

This is how the formula is setup:

$$\frac{DO \times V}{DH}$$

**DO** is what the Physician has ordered

V is from your label on the drug bottle: it stands for how the drug on hand is measured. The above order states there is 500 mg/ml; this "ml" stands for 1 because it is singular. There are 500 mg per 1 ml of solution. The solution is what carries (transports) the drug.

**DH** is the drug on hand, the drug that is in the V that you used. This is the drug on hand in the bottle and in that 1 ml.

Now let's look at the formula in action. How many milliliters do I give?

$$\frac{DO \; 1g \times V \; 1ml}{DH \; 500mg} = 1ml$$

The drug on hand (unit of measurement) always has to match the doctor's order. Never change the doctor's order to match what you have on hand. So the only units that should be changed are those on the bottom of the formula.

Changing the 500 mg to 0.5 gm on the bottom will now change your numbers to the following:

$$\frac{DO \; 1g \times V \; 1ml}{DH \; 0.5 \; g \; (500 \; mg)} = 2ml$$

Starting to make sense?

Let's look at another example using tablets.

The Doctor has ordered 324 mg of Drug A, and you have a pill bottle with a label that reads as follows:

| Drug A |
| :---: |
| 81 mg/tab |
| 200 tablets |

The fact that there are 200 tablets in the bottle is not a concern for our calculations. We want to pay attention to where it states that there is a certain amount of drug to a certain amount of fluid or tablet, and how it is carried. Think of looking for a pair, should always be paired together, a dose and a vehicle.

This is the formula:

$$\frac{DO\ 324mg \times V\ 1tab}{DH\ 81mg} = \underline{\quad} tabs$$

The doctor's order and the drug on hand match (milligram to milligram), so no conversion is needed. The end result is:

$$\frac{324mg \times 1tab}{81\ mg} = 4\ tabs$$

Let's do another. The Doctor has ordered 650 mg of Drug A, and you have a pill bottle with a label that reads as follows:

| Drug A |
| :---: |
| 325 mg/tab |
| 200 tablets |

This is the formula:

$$\frac{DO\ 650mg \times V\ 1tab}{DH\ 325\ mg} = \underline{\quad} tabs$$

The doctor's order and the drug on hand match (milligram to milligram), so no conversion is needed. The end result is:

$$\frac{650 \text{ mg} \times \text{V 1tab}}{325 \text{ mg}} = 2 \text{ tabs}$$

We have finished our first formula, so let's move on to another one. Ready?

The doctor's order is to give a patient 2 mg/kg intravenously (IV) push. This means to give the patient the entire amount of drug at one time through the IV. The patient's weight is 175 lbs. The formula used and the labels of the medication are as follows:

$$\frac{DO \times \text{wt.} \times V}{DH} = \underline{\quad} \text{ml}$$

| Drug A |
| :---: |
| 100 mg/ml |
| 30 ml |

The first step is to convert pounds to kilograms. The patient weighs 175 lbs and there are 2.2 lbs/kg:

175 lbs ÷ 2.2 kg/lb = 79.5 kg (round to 80 kg)

Now that we have the weight, let's set up the formula by filling in the correct numbers:

$$\frac{2 \text{ mg} \times 80 \text{ kg} \times 1 \text{ ml}}{100 \text{ mg}} = 1.6 \text{ ml}$$

You can see from the above label that 30 ml is the total amount of solution in the medication bottle. The 100 mg/1 ml is the pair you are looking for. This means there are 100 mg in every 1 ml of solution; 100 mg is the drug on hand and 1 ml is the vehicle.

Let's do one more formula with the drug on hand being different from the doctor's order:

The doctor's order is to administer 2 mcg/kg of Drug A. The patient's weight is 150 kg. The medication bottle on hand is per the label shown below:

> Drug A
>
> 2 mg/1 ml
>
> 4 mg/2 ml
>
> 30 ml

This label shows several numbers on it, which can be confusing. You are still looking for the pair, as you see there is two pair here: 2 mg/1 ml and 4 mg/ 2ml. You can use either one of these, but you have to use both parts of the pair. If you use 1 ml for the vehicle, then you must use 2 mg for the drug on hand. If you use 2 ml for the vehicle, then you must use 4 mg for the drug on hand. Never mix the measurements for the two pair. Do not use 1 ml as the vehicle and 4 mg as the drug on hand. You will use the wrong calculation, get the wrong answer, and the patient will receive the wrong dosage of medication. The 30 ml at the bottom of the label is the total amount of solution in the bottle. The formula with the correct numbers in place is as follows:

$$\frac{2 \text{ mcg} \times 150 \text{ kg} \times 1 \text{ ml}}{2 \text{ mg}} = \_\_\_\text{ml}$$

What is wrong with this formula? I hope you figured it out. Remember the basic rule: the drug on hand must be the same as the doctor's order. You have to change 2 mg to micrograms. Move the decimal three places to the right and 2 mg becomes 2000 mcg. Let's look at the formula again with the correction:

$$\frac{2 \text{ mcg} \times 150 \text{ kg} \times 1 \text{ ml}}{2000 \text{ mcg}} = 0.15 \text{ ml}$$

Okay, it is time to go to the next formula. So far we have covered how to figure out a patient's medication using pills, a one-time IV push, and a one-time IV push that is weight based. We have changed pounds to kilograms and milligrams to micrograms.

Now we will cover IV infusions. There are some basic rules for working with IV calculations. When orders are written in hours (hr) and liters (L), the hours must be converted to minutes and the liters must be changed to milliliters. An IV infusion is the only time you will convert a doctor's order. Changing liters to milliliters does not change the order as far as what the patient gets. The IV formula is used to figure out how many drops per minute you give the patient when administering the fluid and/or drug that the doctor ordered.

When infusing IV fluids, the IV tubing has different gtt/ml (drops per milliliter) sets. You must look at the drop factor that is on the label of the IV tubing package. For teaching purposes, labels will be given that have different drop factors on them.

Now let's look at an IV formula. In IV formulas, the V stands for Volume. Some people look at it as the doctor's order; either way you will get the right formula.

$$\frac{V \times gtt}{Time}$$

The only two units used on the bottom of the formulas are DH or Time; everything else goes on top.

Let's look at an order: Administer 1.5 L of NS (normal saline) over 4 hr using a 10 gtt factor.

When the numbers are added to the formula this is what it looks like:

$$\frac{1.5 \text{ L} \times 10 \text{ gtt/ml}}{4 \text{ hr}} = \_\_\_ \text{gtt/min}$$

We have to convert some numbers. Liters needs to be changed to milliliters and hours needs to be changed to minutes. Let's look at it with the numbers changed:

$$\frac{1500 \text{ ml} \times 10 \text{ gtt/ml}}{240 \text{ min}} = 62.5 \text{ gtt/min (round to 63 gtt/min)}$$

You have to round the number of drops (gtt) because you can not give half a drop. When the liters and hours are changed, you need to

8

remember there are 1000 ml to 1 L and there are 60 minutes to an hour. Let's look at another one: Administer 250 ml of NS per hour using a 15 gtt factor. Here is the equation:

$$\frac{250 \text{ ml} \times 15 \text{ gtt/ml}}{60 \text{ min}} = 62.5 \text{ gtt/min (round to 63 gtt/min)}$$

Let's look at another IV formula that is based on weight: Administer 20 ml/kg of NS per hour using a 10 gtt factor. The patient's weight is 50 lbs.

First we need to convert pounds to kilograms and hours to minutes:

$$\frac{50 \text{ lb}}{2.2 \text{ kg/lb}} = 22.72 \text{ kg (round to 23 kg)} \quad \text{and} \quad 1 \text{ hr} = 60 \text{ min}$$

This is the formula to use:

$$\frac{V \times wt \times gtt}{hr}$$

Now let's plug in the numbers:

$$\frac{20 \text{ ml} \times 23 \text{ kg} \times 10 \text{ gtt/ml}}{60 \text{ min}} = 76.6 \text{ gtt/min (round to 77 gtt/min)}$$

Here is another one to work out: Administer 10 ml/kg of NS and give over 30 min using a 10 gtt factor. The patient's weight is 20 lbs:

$$\frac{20 \text{ lb}}{2.2 \text{ kg/lb}} = 9.09 \text{ kg (round to 9 kg)}$$

Let's plug in the numbers:

$$\frac{10 \text{ ml} \times 9 \text{ kg} \times 10 \text{ gtt/ml}}{30 \text{ min}} = 30 \text{ gtt/min}$$

Now it is time to move on to other formulas. Let's start with this one as follows:

$$\frac{DO \times V \times gtt}{DH}$$

This is the doctor's order: Administer 1 mg/min of Drug A. You have 2 ml of Drug A available. You also have a 500 ml IV bag of NS. How many drops per minute are you going to give the patient in order to administer this order?

Before starting this formula, there is a basic rule you need to remember prior to figuring out the answer. As stated in the problem, you will be adding 2 ml of Drug A to the IV bag (500 ml) you have on hand. Anytime you increase the size (in volume) of an IV bag by 10% or more, the volume must be added to your math calculation, meaning the IV bag size changes (increases).

Another rule to remember is that when you add a drug to an IV bag and set it up to administer drops per minute (gtt/min), you need to use a 60 drop factor for your IV tubing. The only time you use a different drop factor is when you are given a different drop factor to use.

Okay, let's work the problem out now. These are the labels you have for the IV bag and medication.

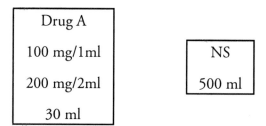

When the doctor's order gives an available amount of a drug, the order will be either the amount of the drug or the volume of liquid you must take out of the medication bottle. If the amount was given in a dosage unit (milligram, microgram, or gram), then you were given the amount of the drug. If the amount was given in milliliters, then you were given the amount of liquid that has been taken out of the bottle.

This problem is giving you the amount of liquid taken out of the bottle, so you have to figure out how much drug is in this liquid in order to figure the correct amount of drops per minute to administer the order.

First you must think about the basic rules to see if they apply. The 10% rule is about changing the volume of an IV bag. You are going to add 2 ml to the 500 ml IV bag. The 2 ml is not 10% of 500 ml, so the IV bag volume does not change. Now we can put our formula together.

You have all the numbers you need for the top of the formula; now you must find the bottom part that is the drug on hand. The drug on hand is the amount of drug inside the available volume that was given to you. Look at the drug label: there are 100 mg to every 1 ml. We need 2 ml taken out of this medication bottle. We know there are 100 mg/1 ml, so it is 2 times 100 mg, which gives you 200 mg. The 200 mg is the drug on hand, now we have everything needed to put the formula together:

| Drug A |
| :---: |
| 100 mg/1 ml |
| 200 mg/2 ml |
| 30 ml |

$$\frac{DO \times V \times gtt}{DH}$$

$$\frac{1 \text{ mg} \times 500 \text{ ml} \times 60 \text{ gtt}}{200 \text{ mg}} = 150 \text{ gtt/min}$$

*Remember the drug on hand units (e.g., milligram, microgram, or gram) have to match the doctor's order. You do not have to change the DH units with this problem. The order was given in milligrams, and the DH was in milligrams.

Let's try another one. This is the doctor's order: Administer 2 mg/min of Drug A. This is what is available: 3 ml of Drug A and an IV bag of NS 200 ml.

| Drug A | NS |
| :---: | :---: |
| 200 mg/1ml | 200 ml |

First look at the volume you are going to take out of the medication bottle. The 3 ml is not 10% of the IV bag of 200 ml, so the volume number does not change.

The only number left to find is the drug on hand (DH). We need 3 ml taken out of the medication bottle. There are 200 mg to every 1 ml, and we need 3 ml. This means we take 3 times 200 mg, which equals 600 mg, so our drug on hand is 600 mg. The DH matches the order, so the milligrams do not have to be changed to any other unit.

Let's do the formula now:

$$\frac{2 \text{ mg} \times 200 \text{ ml} \times 60 \text{ gtt}}{600 \text{ mg}} = 40 \text{ gtt/min}$$

Now let's look at the same formula, but with a change to the volume and DH units. This is the order: Administer 6 mcg/min of Drug A. This is what is available: 15 ml of Drug A and an IV bag of NS 100 ml.

First look at the volume you are going to take out of the medication bottle. The 15 ml is 10% or more of the 100 ml IV bag, so the volume number does change.

The only number left to find is the drug on hand (DH). We need 15 ml taken out of the medication bottle. There is 1 mg to every 1 ml, and we need 15 ml. This means 15 times 1 mg, which equals 15 mg, so our drug on hand is 15 mg. The DH does not match the order, so the milligrams need to be changed to micrograms.

| Drug A | NS |
|---|---|
| 1 mg/1 ml | 100 ml |

Let's do the formula now. This is the formula without the changes:

$$\frac{6 \text{ mcg} \times 100 \text{ ml} \times 60 \text{ gtt}}{15 \text{ mg}}$$

Now let's make the changes: we are adding volume to the IV bag and changing milligrams to micrograms.

$$\frac{6 \text{ mcg} \times 115 \text{ ml} \times 60 \text{ gtt}}{15,000 \text{ mcg}} = 2.76 \text{ gtt (round to 3 gtt/min)}$$

What if the order is based on weight? Let's use the same problem we just finished, but we'll change it to an order based on weight. Order: Administer 6 mcg/kg/min of Drug A. The patient's weight is 150 lbs. This is what is available: 15 ml of Drug A and a 100 ml IV bag.

The weight in pounds must be changed to kilograms:

$$\frac{150 \text{ lbs}}{2.2 \text{ kg/lb}} = 68.16 \text{ kg (round to 68 kg)}$$

First look at the volume you are going to take out of the medication bottle. The 15 ml is 10% or more of the 100 ml IV bag, so the volume number does need to change.

The only number left to plug into the formula is the drug on hand (DH). We need to take 15 ml out of the medication bottle. There is 1 mg to every 1 ml, so there are 15 mg in the 15 ml. The drug on hand is 15 mg. The DH does not match the doctor's order: the milligrams need to be changed to micrograms.

| Drug A | NS |
|---|---|
| 1 mg/1 ml | 100 ml |

Let's do the formula now. This is the formula before any changes:

$$\frac{6 \text{ mcg} \times 68 \text{ kg} \times 100 \text{ ml} \times 60 \text{ gtt}}{15 \text{ mg}}$$

Now let's make the changes: 15 ml are added to the IV bag, and milligrams are changed to micrograms:

$$\frac{6 \text{ mcg} \times 68 \text{ kg} \times 115 \text{ ml} \times 60 \text{ gtt}}{15,000 \text{ mcg}} = 187.68 \text{ gtt (round to 188 gtt/min)}$$

Let's do one more with the weight in the formula. This is the doctor's order: Administer 5 mcg/kg/min of Drug A. The patient's weight is 220 lbs. This is what is available: 20 ml of Drug A and a 250 ml IV bag.

First, the patient's weight must be changed to kilograms:

$$\frac{220 \text{ lbs}}{2.2 \text{ kg/lb}} = 100 \text{ kg}$$

Now look at the volume you are going to take out of the medication bottle. The 20 ml are not 10% or more of the 250 ml IV bag, so the volume number does not change.

The only number left to plug into the formula is the drug on hand (DH). We need 20 ml taken out of the medication bottle. This drug label is different because it is not broken down into how much drug is in every 1 ml. The drug label states there are 250 mg to every 20 ml; we need 20 ml, so the drug on hand is 250 mg. The DH does not match the doctor's orders: the milligrams need to be changed to micrograms.

| Drug A | NS |
|---|---|
| 250 mg/20 ml | 250 ml |

Let's do the formula now. This is the formula before any changes:

$$\frac{5 \text{ mcg} \times 100 \text{ kg} \times 250 \text{ ml} \times 60 \text{ gtt}}{250 \text{ mg}}$$

Now let's change milligrams to micrograms:

$$\frac{5 \text{ mcg} \times 100 \text{ kg} \times 250 \text{ ml} \times 60 \text{ gtt}}{250,000 \text{ mcg}} = 30 \text{ gtt/min}$$

Let's move on to the next type of formula. This one is a little different because the problem requires two steps. You have to use two formulas to solve the problem, but they are formulas that have already been introduced. This is the doctor's order: Administer 1 gm of Drug A over 60 min.

The doctor is asking you to administer a set amount of a drug over a set amount of time. The first step is to find out how much volume you have to take out of the medication bottle to equal the amount of drug ordered. The second part is to infuse the entire volume you have over a set amount of time.

Here are the labels you have:

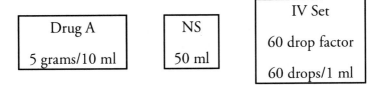

The first step is to find how much volume to remove from the drug bottle. The formula for step one is the same formula you were taught at the beginning of the book:

$$\frac{DO \times V}{DH}$$

Let's fill in this formula with the numbers:

$$\frac{1 \text{ gm} \times 10 \text{ ml}}{5 \text{ gm}} = 2 \text{ ml}$$

A total volume of 2 ml needs to be taken out of the drug bottle to equal the doctor's order. The basic rules still apply: Is the 2 ml amount 10% or more of the volume in the IV bag? No, it is not, so the volume does not change. Are the units the same? The order is in grams and the DH is in grams, so no changes are needed.

The first step is to find out whether or not the IV bag volume is going to change. It doesn't matter if the order is for 1 gm or 100 gm; the dosage is the entire amount that is going to be given over the 60 min. Remember that giving volume to a patient over a period of time is an IV calculation. The IV calculation is the second step to solving the problem. This is the IV formula:

$$\frac{V \times gtt}{Time}$$

Let's fill in the formula:

$$\frac{50 \text{ ml} \times 60 \text{ gtt}}{60 \text{ min}} = 50 \text{ gtt/min}$$

When looking at this type of problem, you must separate it into two steps. First you must look at the drug label to find out how much volume to take out of the bottle that will equal the amount of the drug that you need. After figuring the volume, you need to see if that number is 10% or more of the volume in the IV bag. If it is 10% or more, then the volume of the IV bag will need to change in your IV formula.

Let's look at a problem that shows this increase in volume. This is the doctor's order: Administer 10 gm of Drug A over 60 min.

The doctor is asking you to administer a set amount of a drug over a set amount of time. The first step is to find out how much volume you have to take out of the medication bottle to equal the amount of drug ordered. The second part is to infuse the entire volume you have over a set amount of time.

Here are the labels you have:

| Drug A | NS | IV Set |
|---|---|---|
| 5 gms/10 ml | 50 ml | 60 drop factor |
| | | 60 drops/1ml |

The first step is to find how much volume to remove from the drug bottle:

$$\frac{DO \times V}{DH}$$

Let's fill in this formula with the numbers:

$$\frac{10 \text{ gm} \times 10 \text{ ml}}{5 \text{ gm}} = 20 \text{ ml}$$

A total volume of 20 ml needs to be taken out of the drug bottle to equal the doctor's order. Is the 20 ml amount 10% or more of the IV bag's volume? Yes, it is, so the volume in the formula does need to change. Are the units the same? We have grams in the doctor's order, and our DH is in grams, so the units do not need to change.

16

Remember that the first step is only to find out whether or not the IV bag volume is going to change. The second step is figuring the IV calculation for the formula:

$$\frac{V \times gtt}{Time}$$

Let's fill in the formula, remembering that the volume in the IV bag has increased to 70 ml:

$$\frac{70 \text{ ml} \times 60 \text{ gtt}}{60 \text{ min}} = 70 \text{ gtt/min}$$

The next type of problem is the same as what we just finished, but a weight has been added to the doctor's order: Administer 10 mg/kg of Drug A over 10 min. The patient's weight is 190 lbs.

First, you have to change the pounds to kilograms:

$$\frac{190 \text{ lbs}}{2.2 \text{ kg/lb}} = 86.36 \text{ kg (round to 86 kg)}$$

Here are the labels you have:

| | | |
|---|---|---|
| Drug A | NS | IV Set |
| 50 mg/1 ml | 50 ml | 60 drop factor |
| | | 60 drops/1ml |

The first step is to find how much volume to remove from the drug bottle. Here is the formula with the weight added:

$$\frac{DO \times wt \times V}{DH}$$

Let's fill in this formula with the numbers:

$$\frac{10 \text{ mg} \times 86 \text{ kg} \times 1 \text{ ml}}{50 \text{ mg}} = 17.2 \text{ ml (round to 17 ml)}$$

Now we know a total volume of 17 ml needs to be taken out of the drug bottle to equal the doctor's order. The basic rules still apply. Is the 17 ml amount 10% or more of the 50 ml IV bag? Yes, it is, so the volume does change. Are the units the same? We have milligrams ordered and our DH is in milligrams, so the units do not need to change.

The first step is only to find out whether or not the IV bag volume is going to change. The second step is figuring the IV formula:

$$\frac{V \times gtt}{Time}$$

Let's fill in the formula. The IV bag's volume did increase by 10% or more, so the volume in the formula is now a total of 67 ml:

$$\frac{67\ ml \times 60\ gtt}{10\ min} = 402\ gtt/min$$

*Hint. Here is a hint to help you at times when you can skip step one of the two-step problems we just completed. You have to read the labels closely. I will give you an example.

This is the doctor's order: Administer 5 gm of Drug A over 30 min. Here are the labels you have:

| Drug A | NS | IV Set |
|---|---|---|
| 10 gm/5 ml | 100 ml | 60 drop factor<br>60 drops/1 ml |

The first step is to find how much volume to remove from the drug bottle. The second step is to add the volume to the IV bag if the amount is 10% or more. Look at the IV bag label; you have a 100 ml bag. What is 10% of this bag? It is 10 ml. You would have to take 10 ml or more out of the medication bottle to change your IV bag volume. You do not even have to do the first step because the order of 5 gm is only 2.5 ml, which is less than 10 ml. You can go straight to the IV formula:

$$\frac{100\ ml \times 60\ gtt}{30\ min} = 200\ gtt/min$$

*Guess what? There are only two more formulas to learn, and this will cover the most common formulas used by paramedics.*

The last formulas to learn deal with making concentrations of drugs and then administering the medication to the patient in an IV drip. The first part of the problem is a formula to make the concentration, and the second part of the formula is to figure out how many drops per minute (gtt/min) to give the patient. With this type of problem, there are a few ways to figure the answers. I will share these with you after presenting the basic formula. This last type of problem is sometimes the most confusing because there are a few options for doing the calculations. I will explain the options that are frequently used by paramedics.

*Okay, let's get started!*

This is the doctor's order: Make (Utilize) a 4:1 concentration and administer Drug A at 3 mg/min.

First Step:

1. How many milliliters of the drug will be added to the IV bag? ____ml

   *(This will make the concentration.)*

Second Step:

2. What is the drip rate? ____gtt/min

   *(This will figure out how many drops per minute will equal the order.)*

Here are the labels you have:

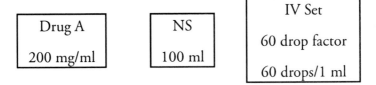

| Drug A | NS | IV Set |
|---|---|---|
| 200 mg/ml | 100 ml | 60 drop factor |
| | | 60 drops/1 ml |

The first step is to find out how much volume to remove from the medication bottle in order to make the concentration ordered.

You are to make a 4:1 concentration; this means you have to add four parts to every one part. In other words, add 4 mg of the drug for every 1 ml in the IV bag you are going to use. If you think about this, it means to multiply the drug concentration by each milliliter in the bag (4 × 100). Let's look at the formula for the first part:

$$\frac{DO \times V \times VH}{DH}$$

In the first part, there are two V's, one stands for the volume and the other stands for the vehicle. To prevent confusion use VH for the vehicle and V for the volume. Another confusing part in the first step is that the DO is the concentration ordered. Let's plug in the numbers:

$$\frac{4 \times 100 \text{ ml} \times 1 \text{ ml}}{200 \text{ mg}} = 2 \text{ ml}$$

The vehicle and the drug on hand are taken from the medication label. Here are the labels again:

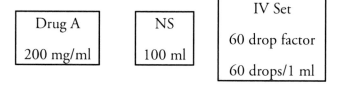

The first answer to the problem is 2 ml. You will add 2 ml of Drug A to the IV bag to make the 4:1 concentration. The 2 ml taken out of the drug bottle will equal 400 mg of Drug A because there are 200 mg to every 1 ml.

Okay, it is time to work out the second part of the problem. Using the same labels, we will have all the numbers we need. The formula is as follows:

$$\frac{DO \times V \times gtt}{DH}$$

When we plug in the numbers, there is one step you must remember: you have made a new drug on hand. In the first part, you figured out the amount of milliliters to take out of the medication bottle to make the concentration; this concentration is the new DH. How much drug is in the 2 ml volume you took out of the bottle? It is 400 mg of Drug A. The new vehicle is the IV bag you added the medication to, which contains 100 ml. These are the numbers you plug into the formula. Now let's do the second part:

$$\frac{3 \text{ mg/min} \times 100 \text{ ml} \times 60 \text{ gtt}}{400 \text{ mg}} = 45 \text{ gtt/min}$$

The 2 ml of drug is not 10% or more of the IV bag, so the volume number does not change. The order is milligrams and the DH is in milligrams, so no changes are needed to the DH.

There is another formula you can use to figure out the second step. The difference is that the V is not used in the top part of the formula, and the concentration ordered is the DH. Let's look at this formula:

$$\frac{DO \times gtt}{\text{concentration}}$$

Let's plug in the numbers:

$$\frac{3 \text{ mg/min} \times 60 \text{ gtt}}{4} = 45 \text{ gtt/min}$$

*Hint. The doctor's order is 3 mg/min, think of the minute part as the drop factor, 60 gtt/ml. How many seconds are there in a minute? Sixty (60). The order's 4:1 is the 4mg:1ml which is the DH (4).

A helpful way to look at this formula is to think about what you are being asked to find. You are trying to find out how much drug you must add to the IV bag to make the concentration that was ordered.

The first step of the original formula (concentration 4:1) is how to find the concentration; the concentration is the DH of the second step. Let me explain what I mean. Look at the problem we just completed. I will show the problem again as follows:

This is the doctor's order: Make (Utilize) a 4:1 concentration and administer 3 mg/min of Drug A.

1. How many milliliters of the drug will be added to the bag? ____ml

2. What is the drip rate? ____gtt/min

Here are the labels you have:

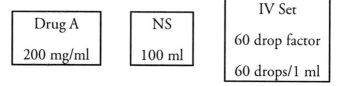

| Drug A | NS | IV Set |
|---|---|---|
| 200 mg/ml | 100 ml | 60 drop factor |
| | | 60 drops/1 ml |

The first step is to find out how much volume to remove from the medication bottle in order to make the concentration.

First Step:

$$\frac{DO \times V \times VH}{DH}$$

$$\frac{4\ mg \times 100\ ml \times 1ml}{200\ mg} = 2\ ml$$

The top part of the equation is how much drug you are going to add to the IV bag to make the 4:1 concentration: 4 mg × 100 ml = 400 mg. This is the same number you will use as the DH in the second step of the formula.

Second Step:

$$\frac{DO \times V \times gtt}{DH}$$

$$\frac{3\ mg/min \times 100\ ml \times 60\ gtt}{400\ mg} = 45\ gtt/min$$

Sometimes you can look at the label in the first step and not even have to go through setting up the first formula. We need 400 mg of the drug to make the concentration, and the first step figures out how many milliliters you have to take out of the medication bottle to get 400 mg. Look at the label. The label states there are 200 mg/ml, so we would need 2 ml to equal the 400 mg. *(If the order was 5:1, we would need 500 mg, which would equal 2.5 ml.)*

*Let's do another problem using a weight and having to change the units (milligrams to micrograms).*

This is the doctor's order: Make (utilize) a 3200:1 concentration and administer at 15 mcg/kg/min of Drug A. The patient's weight is 200 lbs.

Here are the labels you have:

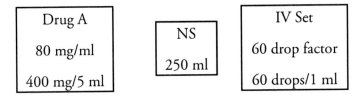

| Drug A<br><br>80 mg/ml<br><br>400 mg/5 ml | NS<br><br>250 ml | IV Set<br><br>60 drop factor<br><br>60 drops/1 ml |

First Step:

1. How many milliliters of the drug will be added to the bag? ____ml

   *(This will make the concentration.)*

Second Step:

2. What is the drip rate ____gtt/min

   *(This will figure out how many drops per minute will equal the order.)*

The weight is 200 lbs. When pounds are converted to kilograms you will get 91 kg:

$$\frac{200 \text{ lbs}}{2.2 \text{ kg/lb}} = 91 \text{ kg}$$

The first step is to find out how much volume to remove from the medication bottle in order to make the concentration ordered. You are to make a 3200:1 concentration; this means you have to add 3200 parts to every one part. In other words, add 3200 mcg of the drug to every 1 ml in the IV bag you are going to use. If you think about this, it means to multiply the drug concentration by each milliliter in the bag (3200 × 250). Let's look at the formula for the first part:

$$\frac{DO \times V \times VH}{DH}$$

Remember, in the first part there are two V's: one stands for the volume, and the other stands for the vehicle. Let's plug in the numbers:

$$\frac{3200 \times 250 \text{ ml} \times 1 \text{ ml}}{80,000 \text{ mcg}} = 10 \text{ ml}$$
(80 mg changed to micrograms)

The vehicle and drug on hand are taken from the medication label. Here are the labels again:

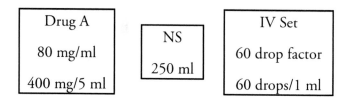

The first answer to the problem is 10 ml. It will take 10 ml of Drug A added to the 250 ml IV bag to make the 3200:1 concentration. The 10 ml taken out of the drug bottle will equal 800 mg of Drug A (remember, you will have to change this to mcg).

Okay, time to work out the second part of the problem. Using the same labels, we will have all the numbers we need. The formula is as follows:

$$\frac{DO \times wt \times V \times gtt}{DH}$$

When we plug in the numbers, there is one step you must remember: you have made a new drug on hand. In the first part, you figured out the amount of milliliters to take out of the medication bottle to make the concentration; the concentration is the new DH. How much drug is in the 10 ml volume you took out of the bottle? It is 800 mg of Drug A. The new vehicle is the 250 ml IV bag. These are the numbers you need to plug into the formula. Let's do the second part:

$$\frac{15 \text{ mcg} \times 91 \text{ kg} \times 250 \text{ ml} \times 60 \text{ gtt}}{800,000 \text{ mcg}} = 25.59 \text{ gtt/min (round to 26 gtt/min)}$$
(800 mg changed to micrograms)

If we look at all the basic rules, the 10ml is not 10% or more of the IV bag, so this number does not change. The order is micrograms and the DH is in milligrams, so we had to change milligrams to micrograms.

If you use the second way shown to figure out concentrations, this is how it would be set up:

First Step:

$$\frac{DO \times V \times VH}{DH}$$

$$\frac{3200 \times 250 \text{ ml} \times 1 \text{ ml}}{80,000 \text{ mcg}} = 10 \text{ ml}$$
$$(80 \text{ mg})$$

Second Step:

$$\frac{DO \times wt \times gtt}{\text{concentration}}$$

$$\frac{15 \text{ mcg} \times 91 \text{ kg} \times 60 \text{ gtt}}{3200} = 26 \text{ gtt/min}$$

I have added one more type of solution to work out concentration formulas that you will see used in the field. There is a method called the *clock method*, but it is only used when making 4:1 concentrations. The clock is used to figure out your drop rate (gtt/min) after making a 4:1 concentration. This is how it works. Think of the front of a clock starting at the fifteen minute spot, which is 3 o'clock. Every fifteen minutes stands for 15 gtt/min with an IV drip. Every fifteen minute increment of the clock stands for an additional 15 gtt/min. The first fifteen minute spot on the clock (15 gtt/min) is the starting point for administering a 4:1 concentration IV drip to a patient, starting at 1 mg/min. The patient gets 1 mg/min, which equals 15 gtt/min. If the doctor orders 2 mg/min, then the patient receives 30 gtt/min, and so on:

1 mg/min = 15 gtt/min

2 mg/min = 30 gtt/min

3 mg/min = 45 gtt/min

4 mg/min = 60 gtt/min

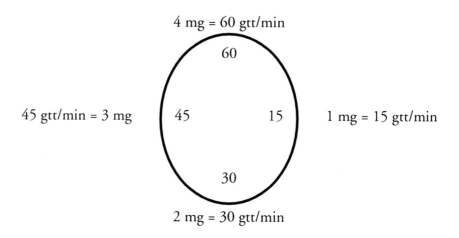

Congratulations you have completed med math!

I have added several practice problems for you, including some med math word problems. While learning med math, you get in the habit of only being able to set up problems using the labels. When you are given a problem in written format without a label, you might become confused, so I have added a few word problems to help you figure out how to set up the problems. The remainder of this book is practice problems.

# Chapter 3
# Med Math Practice
# Word Problems

Administer a Dopamine infusion at 5 mcg/kg/min. The patient weighs 150 lbs. This is what you have available: Dopamine 400 mg in NS 250 ml IV bag. Your infusion rate would be:

$$\frac{5 \text{ mcg} \times 68 \text{ kg} \times 250 \text{ ml} \times 60 \text{ gtt}}{400,000 \text{ mcg}}$$
$$(400 \text{ mg})$$

Answer: 13 gtt/min

Administer a Nitro infusion at 3 mcg/min using a 5:1 concentration. You are using a NS 100 ml bag.

A. The Nitro label indicates 1 mg/ml. How many milliliters of Nitro would you add to the bag? ___ml

$$\frac{5 \times 100 \text{ml} \times 1 \text{ml}}{1000 \text{ mcg}} = 0.5 \text{ ml}$$
$$(1 \text{ mg changed to DO units})$$

B. What is your infusion rate using a microdrip infusion set?

$$\frac{3 \text{ mcg} \times 100 \text{ ml} \times 60 \text{ gtt}}{500 \text{ mcg}} = \text{Answer 36 gtt/min}$$

Or

$$\frac{3 \text{ mcg} \times 60 \text{ gtt}}{5} = 36 \text{ gtt/min}$$

You are ordered to administer Amiodarone 2 mg/kg to a patient who weighs 100 lbs. Available is Amiodarone 100 mg/5 ml. How many milliliters would you administer?

100 lb/2.2 kg = 45 kg      100 lb/2 kg = 50 kg – 10% (5) = 45 kg

$$\frac{2 \text{ mg} \times 45 \text{ kg} \times 5 \text{ ml}}{100 \text{ mg}} = \text{Answer 4.5 ml}$$

Infuse Amiodarone 150 mg over 10 min. Amiodarone comes 150 mg in 3 ml, and your patient weighs 300 lbs. Mix the drug in a 50 ml bag of $D_5W$ and infuse using a 60 gtt/ml infusion set. What is your infusion rate?

$$\frac{50 \text{ ml} \times 60 \text{ gtt}}{10 \text{ min}} = 300 \text{ gtt/min}$$

Infuse Amiodarone 150 mg over 10 minutes. Amiodarone comes 150 mg in 10 ml and your patient weighs 100 lbs. Mix the drug in a 100 ml bag of $D_5W$ and infuse using a 10 gtt/ml infusion set. What is your infusion rate?

$$\frac{110 \text{ ml} \times 10 \text{ gtt}}{10 \text{ min}} = 110 \text{ gtt/min}$$

Administer a Nitro infusion at 4 mcg/min using a 3:1 concentration. You are using a NS 100 ml bag.

A. The Nitro label indicates 1 mg/ml. How many ml of Nitro would you add to the bag?

3 mcg × 100 ml = 300 mcg = 0.3 mg = 0.3 ml

Or

$$\frac{3 \text{ mcg} \times 100 \text{ ml} \times 1 \text{ ml}}{1000 \text{ mcg}}$$
$$(1 \text{ mg})$$

B. What is your infusion rate using a microdrip infusion set?

$$\frac{4 \text{ mcg} \times 100 \text{ ml} \times 60 \text{ gtt}}{300 \text{ mcg}} = 80 \text{ gtt/min}$$

Or

$$\frac{4 \text{ mcg} \times 60 \text{ gtt}}{3} = 80 \text{ gtt/min}$$

You are ordered to administer Amiodarone 4 mg/kg to a patient who weighs 150 lbs. Available is Amiodarone 100 mg/10 ml. How many milliliters would you administer?

150 lb/2.2 kg = 68 kg     150 lbs/2 kg = 75 kg – 10% = 68 kg (67.5)

$$\frac{4 \text{ mg} \times 68 \text{ kg} \times 10 \text{ ml}}{100 \text{ mg}} = 27 \text{ ml}$$

Administer a Dopamine infusion at 5 mcg/kg/min. The patient weighs 200 pounds. Use Dopamine 400 mg in 250 ml IV bag. What would be your infusion rate?

$$\frac{5 \text{ mcg} \times 91 \text{ kg} \times 250 \text{ ml} \times 60 \text{ gtt}}{400,000 \text{ mcg}}$$     or     $$\frac{5 \text{ mcg} \times 91 \text{ kg} \times 60}{1600 \text{ mcg}}$$
$$(400 \text{ mg})$$                                     (concentration)

Answer: 17 gtt/min

With this problem you are not given the concentration to make. You are given the amount of drug to add to the IV bag to make the concentration the physician wants. How do you figure out what this concentration is? To find the concentration of a drug in a volume, take the drug amount and divide by the volume:

$$\frac{D}{V}$$

In the previous problem, this is how to figure the concentration:

$$\frac{D\ \ 400\ mg}{V\ \ 250\ ml} = 1.6\ mg/ml$$

The 1.6 mg concentration needs to be changed to the DO unit of measurement, milligrams to micrograms. 1.6 mg = 1600 mcg. 1600 mcg is the concentration. You will frequently use standard concentrations of drugs and IV solution out in the field. You may work in a place that only mixes Dopamine 800 mg in a 250 ml IV bag, which will give you a 3200 mcg/ml concentration. This means you would use the same formula all the time when you use this standard combination of drug and concentration.

# Chapter 4
# Med Math Practice Problems

The next practice problems will be set up using labels and will include all the formulas you have learned. The answers are in the back of the book at the end of the practice problems.

Good Luck!

1. Order: Administer 324 mg of Aspirin
How many tablets do you give? _____tab

| Aspirin |
| --- |
| 81 mg/tablet |

2. Order: Administer 1000 mg of Tylenol
How many tablets do you give? _____tab

| Tylenol |
| --- |
| 500 mg/tablet |

3. Order: Administer 300 mg of Motrin
How many tablets do you give? _____tab

| Motrin |
| --- |
| 200 mg/tablet |

4. Order: Administer 2 mg of Narcan IV
How many milliliters do you give? _____ml

> Narcan
> 2 mg/ml

5. Order: Administer 2 mg of Versed IV
How many milliliters do you give? _____ml

> Versed
> 5 mg/ml

6. Order: Administer 5 mg of Valium IV
How many milliliters do you give? _____ml

> Valium
> 10 mg/2 ml
> 5 mg/1 ml

7. Order: Administer 1gm of Calcium Chloride IV
How many milliliters do you give? _____ml

> Calcium Chloride
> 100 mg/1 ml

8. Order: Administer 2 mg of Atropine IV
How many milliliters do you give? _____ml

> Atropine
> 0.1 mg/ml

9. Order: Administer 1 mg/kg of Lidocaine IV
Patient's weight: 80 kg
How many milliliters do you give? _____ml

> Lidocaine
> 100 mg/5 ml

10. Order: Administer 5 mg/kg of Bretylium IV
Patient's weight: 80 kg
How many milliliters do you give?_____ml

> Bretylium
> 50 mg/1 ml

11. Order: Administer 2 mg/kg of Lasix IV
Patient's weight: 150 lbs
How many milliliters do you give?____ml

| Lasix |
|---|
| 10 mg/1 ml |

12. Order: Administer 1 mg/kg of Benadryl IV
Patient's weight: 55 lbs
How many milliliters do you give? ____ml

| Benadryl |
|---|
| 50 mg/1 ml |

13. Order: Administer 0.2 mg/kg of Valium IV
Patient's weight: 50 kg
How many milliliters do you give? ____ml

| Valium |
|---|
| 10 mg/2 ml |

14. Order: Infuse 500 ml of NS over 2 hr
Drop factor 10 gtt/ml
How many drops per minute are you going to give? ____gtt/min

15. Order: Infuse 1 Liter of NS over 6 hr
Drop factor 10 gtt/ml
How many drops per minute are you going to give? ____gtt/min

16. Order: Infuse 30 ml of NS per hour
Drop factor 10 gtt/ml
How many drops per minute are you going to give? ____gtt/min

17. Order: Infuse 200 ml of NS over 30 min
Drop factor 10 gtt/ml
How many drops per minute are you going to give? ____gtt/min

18. Order: Infuse 75 ml of NS over 30 min
Drop factor 15 gtt/ml
How many drops per minute are you going to give? ____gtt/min

19. Order: Infuse 20 ml/kg of NS over 30 min
Drop factor 15 gtt/ml
Patient's weight: 50 kg
How many drops per minute are you going to give? ____gtt/min

20. Order: Infuse 30 ml/kg of NS over 1 hr
Drop factor 10 gtt/ml
Patient's weight: 60 kg
How many drops per minute are you going to give? _____gtt/min

21. Order: Infuse 10 ml/kg of NS over 1 hr
Drop factor 10 gtt/ml
Patient's weight: 15 kg
How many drops per minute are you going to give? _____gtt/min

22. Order: Infuse 20 ml/kg of NS over 2 hour
Drop factor 10 gtt/ml
Patient's weight: 33 lbs
How many drops per minute are you going to give? _____gtt/min

23. Order: Infuse 50 ml/kg of NS over 4 hr
Drop factor 10 gtt/ml
Patient's weight: 150 lbs
How many drops per minute are you going to give? _____gtt/min

24. Order: Administer Isuprel 3 mcg/min
Utilize: 10 ml of Isuprel in a 250 ml bag of NS
How many drops per minute do you give? _____gtt/min

| Isuprel | NS |
|---|---|
| 1 mg/10 ml | 250 ml |

25. Order: Administer Lidocaine 4 mg/min
Utilize: 5 ml of Lidocaine in a 250 ml bag of NS
How many drops per minute do you give? _____gtt/min

| Lidocaine | NS |
|---|---|
| 200 mg/1 ml | 250 ml |

26. Order: Administer Epinephrine
6 mcg/min
Utilize: 10 ml of Epinephrine in a
100 ml
bag of NS
How many drops per minute
do you give? _____gtt/min

| Epinephrine | | NS |
| 1 mg/1 ml | | 100 ml |
| 1:1000 | | |

27. Order: Administer Procainamide
2 mg/min
Utilize: 1 ml of Procainamide in a
500 ml
bag of NS
How many drops per minute
do you give? _____gtt/min

| Procainamide | | NS |
| 500 mg/1 ml | | 500 ml |

28. Order: Administer Dopamine 8
mcg/kg/min
Patient's weight: 200 lbs
Utilize: 5 ml of Dopamine in a 250 ml
bag of NS
How many drops per minute
do you give _____gtt/min

| Dopamine | | NS |
| 80 mg/1 ml | | 250 ml |
| 400 mg/5 ml | | |

29. Order: Administer Dopamine 6
mcg/kg/min
Patient's weight: 160 lbs
Utilize: 5 ml of Dopamine in a 100 ml
bag of NS
How many drops per minute
do you give? _____gtt/min

| Dopamine | | NS |
| 80 mg/1 ml | | 100 ml |
| 400 mg/5 ml | | |

30. Order: Administer Dobutamine 4 mcg/kg/min
Patient's weight: 160 lbs
Utilize: 20 ml of Dobutamine in a 500 ml
bag of NS
How many drops per minute
do you give? _____gtt/min

| Dobutamine | NS |
|---|---|
| 250 mg/20 ml | 500 ml |

31. Order: Administer Dobutamine 6 mcg/kg/min
Patient's weight: 220 lbs
Utilize: 20 ml of Dobutamine in a 250 ml
bag of NS
How many drops per minute
do you give? _____gtt/min

| Dobutamine | NS |
|---|---|
| 250 mg/20 ml | 250 ml |

32. Order: Administer Bretylium 6 mg/kg/min
over 20 min
Patient's weight: 190 lbs
IV drop Factor 60 gtt/ml
How many drops per minute
do you give? _____gtt/min

| Bretylium | NS |
|---|---|
| 50 mg/1 ml | 50 ml |

33. Order: Administer Magnesium Sulfate 2 gm
over 40 min
IV drop Factor 60 gtt/ml
How many drops per minute
do you give? _____gtt/min

| Magnesium Sulfate | NS |
|---|---|
| 5 gm/10 ml | 50 ml |

34. Order: Administer Bretylium
10 mg/kg/min
over 10 min
Patient's weight: 150 lbs
IV drop Factor 60 gtt/ml
How many drops per minute
do you give? _____gtt/min

| Bretylium 50 mg/1 ml | NS 50 ml |

35. Order: Administer Magnesium
Sulfate 1 gm
over 30 min
IV drop Factor 60 gtt/ml
How many drops per minute
do you give? _____gtt/min

| Magnesium Sulfate 5 gm/10 ml | NS 50 ml |

36. Order: Administer Lidocaine 2 mg/min
Utilize (make): 4:1 concentration
a.How many milliliters do you add
to the IV bag? _____ml
b.How many drops per minute
do you give? _____gtt/min

| Lidocaine 200 mg/ml | NS 100 ml |

37. Order: Administer Lidocaine 4 mg/min
Utilize (make): 4:1 concentration
a.How many milliliters do you add
to the IV bag? _____ml
b.How many drops per minute
do you give? _____gtt/min

| Lidocaine 200 mg/ml | NS 100 ml |

38. Order: Administer Dopamine
6 mcg/kg/min
Patient's weight: 150 lbs
Utilize (make): 1600:1 concentration
a.How many milliliters
do you add to the IV bag? _____ml
b.How many drops per minute
do you give? _____gtt/min

| Dopamine | NS |
| --- | --- |
| 80 mg/1 ml | 250 ml |
| 400 mg/5 ml | |

39. Order: Administer Dopamine
12 mcg/kg/min
Patient's weight: 200 lbs
Utilize (make): 3200:1 concentration
a.How many milliliters do you add
to the IV bag? _____ml
b.How many drops per minute
do you give? _____gtt/min

| Dopamine | NS |
| --- | --- |
| 80 mg/1 ml | 250 ml |
| 400 mg/5 ml | |

40. Order: Administer Epinephrine
2 mcg/min
Utilize (make): 4:1 concentration
a.How many milliliters do you add
to the IV bag? _____ml
b.How many drops per minute
do you give? _____gtt/min

| Epinephrine | NS |
| --- | --- |
| 1 mg/ml | 100 ml |
| 1:1000 | |

41. Order: Administer Dobutamine
8mcg/kg/min
Patient's weight: 175 lbs
Utilize (make): 500:1 concentration
a.How many milliliters do you add
to the IV bag? _____ml
b.How many drops per minute
do you give? _____gtt/min

| Dobutamine | NS |
| --- | --- |
| 250 mg/20 ml | 250 ml |

42. Order: Administer Dobutamine
15 mcg/kg/min
Patient's weight: 180 lbs
Utilize (make): 500:1 concentration
a.How many milliliters do you add
to the IV bag? ____ml
b.How many drops per minute
do you give? ____gtt/min

| Dobutamine | NS |
|---|---|
| 250 mg/20 ml | 250 ml |

# Appendix
# Answers to Problems

| 1 | 4 tablets | $\dfrac{DO \times V}{DH}$ | $\dfrac{324 \text{ mg} \times 1 \text{ tab}}{81 \text{ mg}}$ |
|---|---|---|---|
| 2 | 2 tablets | $\dfrac{DO \times V}{DH}$ | $\dfrac{100 \text{ mg} \times 1 \text{ tab}}{500 \text{ mg}}$ |
| 3 | 1.5 tablets | $\dfrac{DO \times V}{DH}$ | $\dfrac{300 \text{ mg} \times 1 \text{ tab}}{200 \text{ mg}}$ |
| 4 | 1 ml | $\dfrac{DO \times V}{DH}$ | $\dfrac{2 \text{ mg} \times 1 \text{ ml}}{2 \text{ mg}}$ |
| 5 | 0.4 ml | $\dfrac{DO \times V}{DH}$ | $\dfrac{2 \text{ mg} \times 1 \text{ ml}}{5 \text{ mg}}$ |
| 6 | 1 ml | $\dfrac{DO \times V}{DH}$ | $\dfrac{5 \text{ mg} \times 1 \text{ ml}}{5 \text{ mg}}$ |
| 7 | 10 ml | $\dfrac{DO \times V}{DH}$ | $\dfrac{1 \text{ gm} \times 1 \text{ ml}}{\substack{0.1 \text{ gm} \\ (100 \text{ mg})}}$ |
| 8 | 20 ml | $\dfrac{DO \times V}{DH}$ | $\dfrac{2 \text{ mg} \times 1 \text{ ml}}{0.1 \text{ mg}}$ |
| 9 | 4 ml | $\dfrac{DO \times wt \times V}{DH}$ | $\dfrac{1 \text{ mg} \times 80 \text{ kg} \times 5 \text{ ml}}{100 \text{ mg}}$ |
| 10 | 8 ml | $\dfrac{DO \times wt \times V}{DH}$ | $\dfrac{5 \text{ mg} \times 80 \text{ kg} \times 1 \text{ ml}}{50 \text{ mg}}$ |

| | | | |
|---|---|---|---|
| 11 | 13.6 ml | $\dfrac{\text{DO} \times \text{wt} \times \text{V}}{\text{DH}}$ | $\dfrac{2 \text{ mg} \times 68 \text{ kg} \times 1 \text{ ml}}{10 \text{ mg}}$ |
| 12 | 0.5 ml | $\dfrac{\text{DO} \times \text{wt} \times \text{V}}{\text{DH}}$ | $\dfrac{1 \text{ mg} \times 25 \text{ kg} \times 1 \text{ ml}}{50 \text{ mg}}$ |
| 13 | 2 ml | $\dfrac{\text{DO} \times \text{wt} \times \text{V}}{\text{DH}}$ | $\dfrac{0.2 \text{ mg} \times 50 \text{ kg} \times 2 \text{ ml}}{10 \text{ mg}}$ |
| 14 | 41.6 gtt/ min (round to 42 gtt/ min) | $\dfrac{\text{V} \times \text{gtt}}{\text{Time}}$ | $\dfrac{500 \text{ ml} \times 10 \text{ gtt/ml}}{120 \text{ min}}$ |
| 15 | 27.7 gtt/ min (round to 28 gtt/ min) | $\dfrac{\text{V} \times \text{gtt}}{\text{Time}}$ | $\dfrac{1000 \text{ ml} \times 10 \text{ gtt/ml}}{360 \text{ min}}$ |
| 16 | 5 gtt/min | $\dfrac{\text{V} \times \text{gtt}}{\text{Time}}$ | $\dfrac{30 \text{ ml} \times 10 \text{ gtt/ml}}{60 \text{ min}}$ |
| 17 | 66.6 gtt/ min (round to 67 gtt/ min) | $\dfrac{\text{V} \times \text{gtt}}{\text{Time}}$ | $\dfrac{200 \text{ ml} \times 10 \text{ gtt/ml}}{30 \text{ min}}$ |
| 18 | 37.5 gtt/ min (round to 38 gtt/min | $\dfrac{\text{V} \times \text{gtt}}{\text{Time}}$ | $\dfrac{75 \text{ ml} \times 15 \text{ gtt/ml}}{30 \text{ min}}$ |
| 19 | 500 gtt/ min | $\dfrac{\text{V} \times \text{wt} \times \text{gtt}}{\text{Time}}$ | $\dfrac{20 \text{ ml} \times 50 \text{ kg} \times 15 \text{ gtt/ml}}{30 \text{ min}}$ |
| 20 | 300 gtt/ min | $\dfrac{\text{V} \times \text{wt} \times \text{gtt}}{\text{Time}}$ | $\dfrac{30 \text{ ml} \times 60 \text{ kg} \times 10 \text{ gtt/ml}}{60 \text{ min}}$ |
| 21 | 25 gtt/min | $\dfrac{\text{V} \times \text{wt} \times \text{gtt}}{\text{Time}}$ | $\dfrac{10 \text{ ml} \times 15 \text{ kg} \times 10 \text{ gtt/ml}}{60 \text{ min}}$ |
| 22 | 25 gtt/min | $\dfrac{\text{V} \times \text{wt} \times \text{gtt}}{\text{Time}}$ | $\dfrac{20 \text{ ml} \times 15 \text{ kg} \times 10 \text{ gtt/ml}}{120 \text{ min}}$ |
| 23 | 141.6 gtt/ min (round to 142 gtt/ min) | $\dfrac{\text{V} \times \text{wt} \times \text{gtt}}{\text{Time}}$ | $\dfrac{50 \text{ ml} \times 68 \text{ kg} \times 10 \text{ gtt/ml}}{240 \text{ min}}$ |
| 24 | 45 gtt/min | $\dfrac{\text{V} \times \text{wt} \times \text{gtt}}{\text{Time}}$ | $\dfrac{50 \text{ ml} \times 68 \text{ kg} \times 10 \text{ gtt/ml}}{1000 \text{ mcg}}$ (1 mg) |

| 25 | 60 gtt/min | $\dfrac{DO \times V \times gtt}{DH}$ | $\dfrac{4 \text{ mg} \times 250 \text{ ml} \times 60 \text{ gtt/ml}}{1000 \text{ mg}}$ |
|---|---|---|---|
| 26 | 3.96 gtt/min (round to 4 gtt/min | $\dfrac{DO \times V \times gtt}{DH}$ | $\dfrac{6 \text{ mcg} \times 110 \text{ ml} \times 60 \text{ gtt/ml}}{10,000 \text{ mcg}}$ (10mg) |
| 27 | 120 gtt/min | $\dfrac{DO \times V \times gtt}{DH}$ | $\dfrac{2 \text{ mg} \times 500 \text{ ml} \times 60 \text{ gtt/ml}}{500 \text{ mg}}$ |
| 28 | 27.3 gtt/min (round to 27) | $\dfrac{DO \times wt \times V \times gtt}{DH}$ | $\dfrac{8 \text{ mcg} \times 91 \text{ kg} \times 250 \text{ ml} \times 60 \text{ gtt/ml}}{400,000 \text{ mcg}}$ (400 mg) |
| 29 | 6.57 gtt/min (round to 7) | $\dfrac{DO \times wt \times V \times gtt}{DH}$ | $\dfrac{6 \text{ mcg} \times 73 \text{ kg} \times 100 \text{ ml} \times 60 \text{ gtt/ml}}{400,000 \text{ mcg}}$ (400 mg) |
| 30 | 35 gtt/min | $\dfrac{DO \times wt \times V \times gtt}{DH}$ | $\dfrac{4 \text{ mcg} \times 73 \text{ kg} \times 500 \text{ ml} \times 60 \text{ gtt/ml}}{250,000 \text{ mcg}}$ (250 mg) |
| 31 | 36 gtt/min | $\dfrac{DO \times wt \times V \times gtt}{DH}$ | $\dfrac{6 \text{ mcg} \times 100 \text{ kg} \times 250 \text{ ml} \times 60 \text{ gtt/ml}}{250,000 \text{ mcg}}$ (250 mg) |
| 32 | 180 gtt/min | Step #1 $\dfrac{DO \times wt \times V}{DH}$ | $\dfrac{6 \text{ mg} \times 86 \text{ kg} \times 1 \text{ ml}}{50 \text{ mg}} = 10.32 \text{ ml (10 ml)}$ |
|  |  | Step #2 $\dfrac{V \times gtt}{Time}$ | $\dfrac{60 \text{ ml} \times 60 \text{ gtt/ml}}{20 \text{ min}} = 180 \text{ gtt/min}$ |
| 33 | 75 gtt/min | Step #1 $\dfrac{DO \times V}{DH}$ | $\dfrac{2 \text{ gm} \times 10 \text{ ml}}{5 \text{ gm}} = 4 \text{ ml}$ |
|  |  | Step #2 $\dfrac{V \times gtt}{Time}$ | $\dfrac{50 \times 60 \text{ gtt/ml}}{40 \text{ min}} = 75 \text{ gtt/min}$ |
| 34 | 384 gtt/min | Step #1 $\dfrac{DO \times wt \times V}{DH}$ | $\dfrac{10 \text{ mg} \times 68 \text{ kg} \times 1 \text{ ml}}{50 \text{ mg}} = 13.6 \text{ ml (14 ml)}$ |
|  |  | Step #2 $\dfrac{V \times gtt}{Time}$ | $\dfrac{64 \times 60 \text{ gtt/ml}}{10 \text{ min}} = 384 \text{ gtt/min}$ |
| 35 | 100 gtt/min | Step #1 $\dfrac{DO \times V}{DH}$ | $\dfrac{1 \text{ gm} \times 10 \text{ ml}}{5 \text{ gm}} = 2 \text{ ml}$ |
|  |  | Step #2 $\dfrac{V \times gtt}{Time}$ | $\dfrac{50 \times 60 \text{ gtt/ml}}{30 \text{ min}} = 100 \text{ gtt/min}$ |

**36**  #1  2 ml
#2  30 gtt/ min

Step #1
$$\frac{\text{concentration} \times V \times VH}{DH}$$

$$\frac{4 \text{ mg} \times 100 \text{ ml} \times 1 \text{ ml}}{200 \text{ mg}} = 2 \text{ ml}$$

Step #2
$$\frac{DO \times V \times gtt}{DH}$$

$$\frac{2 \text{ mg} \times 100 \text{ ml} \times 60 \text{ gtt}}{400 \text{ mg}} = 30 \text{ gtt/min}$$

Or
Step #2
$$\frac{DO \times gtt}{\text{concentration}}$$

$$\frac{2 \text{ mg} \times 60 \text{ gtt}}{4}$$

**37**  #1  2 ml
#2  60 gtt/ min

Step #1
$$\frac{\text{concentration} \times V \times VH}{DH}$$

$$\frac{4 \text{ mg} \times 100 \text{ ml} \times 1 \text{ ml}}{200 \text{ mg}} = 2 \text{ ml}$$

Step #2
$$\frac{DO \times V \times gtt}{DH}$$

$$\frac{4 \text{ mg} \times 100 \text{ ml} \times 60}{400 \text{ mg}} = 30 \text{ gtt/min}$$

Or
Step #2
$$\frac{DO \times gtt}{\text{concentration}}$$

$$\frac{4 \text{ mg} \times 60 \text{ gtt}}{4}$$

**38**  #1  5 ml
#2  15 gtt/ min

Step #1
$$\frac{\text{concentration} \times V \times VH}{DH}$$

$$\frac{1600 \text{ mcg} \times 250 \text{ ml} \times 1 \text{ ml}}{80,000 \text{ mcg}} = 5 \text{ ml}$$
(80 mg)

Step #2
$$\frac{DO \times wt \times V \times gtt}{DH}$$

$$\frac{6 \text{ mcg} \times 68 \text{ kg} \times 250 \text{ ml} \times 60 \text{ gtt}}{400,000 \text{ mcg}} = 15.3 \text{ gtt/min}$$
(round to 15 gtt/min)
(400mg)

Or
Step #2
$$\frac{DO \times wt \times gtt}{\text{concentration}}$$

$$\frac{6 \text{ mcg} \times 68 \times 60 \text{ gtt}}{1600}$$

**39**  #1  10 ml
#2  20 gtt/ min

Step #1
$$\frac{\text{concentration} \times V \times VH}{DH}$$
Step #2
$$\frac{DO \times wt \times V \times gtt}{DH}$$

$$\frac{3200 \text{ mcg} \times 250 \text{ ml} \times 1 \text{ ml}}{80,000 \text{ mcg}} = 10 \text{ ml}$$
(80 mg)

$$\frac{12 \text{ mcg} \times 91 \text{ kg} \times 250 \text{ ml} \times 60 \text{ gtt}}{800,000 \text{ mcg}} = 20.47 \text{ gtt/min}$$
(round to 20 gtt/min)
(800 mg)

Or
Step #2
$$\frac{DO \times wt \times gtt}{\text{concentration}}$$

$$\frac{12 \text{ mcg} \times 91 \text{ kg} \times 60 \text{ gtt}}{3200}$$

40   #1  0.4 ml

      #2  30 gtt/ min

Step #1

$$\frac{\text{concentration} \times V \times VH}{DH}$$

Step #2

$$\frac{DO \times V \times gtt}{DH}$$

$$\frac{4 \text{ mcg} \times 100 \text{ ml} \times 1 \text{ ml}}{1000 \text{ mcg}} = 0.4 \text{ ml}$$
$$(1 \text{ mg})$$

$$\frac{2 \text{ mcg} \times 100 \text{ ml} \times 60 \text{ gtt}}{400 \text{ mcg}} = 30 \text{ gtt/min}$$
$$(0.4 \text{ mg})$$

Or

Step #2

$$\frac{DO \times gtt}{\text{concentration}}$$

$$\frac{2 \text{ mcg} \times 60 \text{ gtt}}{4}$$

41   #1  10 ml

      #2  77 gtt/ min

Step #1

$$\frac{\text{concentration} \times V \times VH}{DH}$$

Step #2

$$\frac{DO \times wt \times V \times gtt}{DH}$$

$$\frac{500 \text{ mcg} \times 250 \text{ ml} \times 20 \text{ ml}}{250,000 \text{ mcg}} = 10 \text{ ml}$$
$$(250\text{mg})$$

$$\frac{8 \text{ mcg} \times 80 \text{ kg} \times 250 \text{ ml} \times 60 \text{ gtt}}{125,000 \text{ mcg}} = 76.8 \text{ gtt/min}$$
            (round to 77 gtt/min)
$$(125 \text{ mg})$$

Or

Step #2

$$\frac{DO \times wt \times gtt}{\text{concentration}}$$

$$\frac{8 \text{ mcg} \times 80 \times 60 \text{ gtt}}{500}$$

42   #1  10 ml

      #2  148 gtt/min

Step #1

$$\frac{\text{concentration} \times V \times VH}{DH}$$

Step #2

$$\frac{DO \times wt \times V \times gtt}{DH}$$

Or

Step #2

$$\frac{DO \times wt \times gtt}{\text{concentration}}$$

$$\frac{500 \text{ mcg} \times 250 \text{ ml} \times 20 \text{ ml}}{250,000 \text{ mcg}} = 10 \text{ ml}$$
$$(250 \text{ mg})$$

$$\frac{15 \text{ mcg} \times 82 \text{ kg} \times 250 \text{ ml} \times 60 \text{ gtt}}{125,000 \text{ mcg}} = 147.6 \text{ gtt/min}$$
            (round to 148 gtt/min)
$$(125 \text{ mg})$$

$$\frac{15 \text{ mcg} \times 82 \times 60 \text{ gtt}}{500}$$

CPSIA information can be obtained
at www.ICGtesting.com
Printed in the USA
FFOW03n1924151217
44118934-43415FF